Grandma's Herbal remedies 2 - The secret recipes

by A.H Smithers

Table of Contents

1. Introduction

After the past year compiling several books with my Nan (*Grandma's Herbal Remedies, Grandma's Natural Cleaning and Stain Removal Secrets, and Grandma's Guide to Raising Chickens*), we had come to a crossroads.

Phone Conversation:

Grandma: "That's it, Anton. You have had the best of me. I am done with book publishing."

Anton: "But, Nan, people love your old-worldly, cost saving, and natural living way of life – it should be documented."

Grandma: "I don't think I have anything more to say, or teach! Anyway, I must go as I need to do my oil pulling."

Anton: "This is what I am talking about! What on earth is 'oil pulling'?"

So here we are, for what **WE PROMISE** (she made me write this in bold) will be the very last of the Grandma series. In this book, we cover, in more detail, the final herbal and homemade remedies, as well as a few other interesting techniques for staying healthy – and of course, Oil Pulling!
Herbal remedies have been around for centuries and were the first forms of medicine for early humans. Plants, fruits, tree bark, and flowers were used to treat

everything from minor skin cuts to major infections and viruses.

Today, herbal remedies can offer affordable treatments for common and non-severe illnesses, including diarrhoea, anxiety, depression, stress, bladder, kidney, stomach and intestinal ailments, acne, dry skin, psoriasis, eczema, wound care, water retention, colds, the flu, and headaches.

In this book, we look at a lot less remedies. However, the ones we do look at, it is in far more detail with a lot more recipes and a lot more detail.

To avoid confusion, I have listed the herbs and spices in alphabetical order.

As well as the details about the spices, I also look at Origins/history. How the spice or herb can help a particular ailment, **how it's used**, and how you would make the remedy. I also look at how you would go about growing it, and how easy this is to achieve as well as any **Warnings** that should be adhered to. We also look at the new section recipes.

2. Bishop's Weed

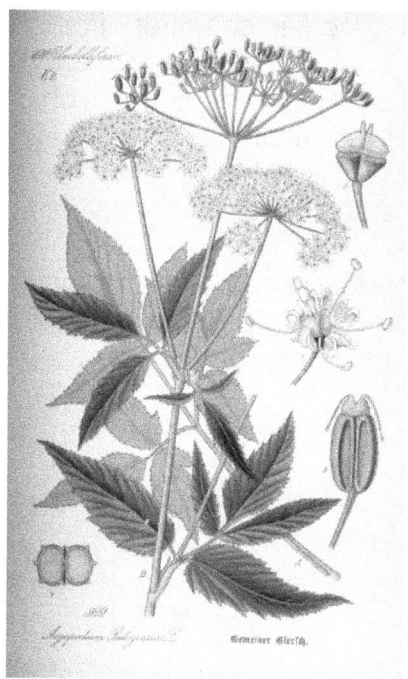

Origins

Bishop's Weed was first discovered centuries ago in India. It was touted as a potent aphrodisiac and used to cure a wide variety of stomach and intestinal illnesses. New mothers used the ground seeds to help relieve colic in babies and dysentery in babies, children, and adults.

Bishop's weed was also used in early modern medicine to relieve asthma and respiratory distress. To create the medicine, the seeds were dried and ground and put into capsules. Today, Bishop's Weed has been replaced by other asthma medications, but it can still be used to treat asthma when used as a herbal remedy.

Ailments

Bishop's Weed helps alleviate symptoms of psoriasis and dry, scaly skin, when directly applied to the skin via an ointment. When consumed internally, it helps with kidney function, bladder infections, chest pain, asthma, and stomach ailments.

How It's Used

The seeds are typically ground or chewed to relieve intestinal discomfort and asthma or brewed into a tea. For the skin, the seeds are infused with a carrier oil or petroleum jelly and applied directly on the skin.

Recipes

Bishop's Weed Seeds

1/2 Cup Seeds
Mortar And Pestle Or Food Processor

Wash the seeds thoroughly and lay them out on a clean towel in a place that will not be disturbed for 72 hours. After 72 hours, the seeds should be completely dry. If you suspect the seeds are not dry, leave them sit for another day.

Place the dried seeds in the mortar and grind them with the pestle until they are completely crushed into a fine powder. Alternatively, you can place the seeds in a food processor and process them for a few seconds. Put the powder into a sterile glass jar and seal with the lid. The powder can be consumed by itself or put into tea or oil. To take by mouth, scoop out one teaspoon and consume. It is not recommended to take more than one teaspoon at a time because the powder is very dry and may result in choking. After consuming, drink a full glass of water to rinse the mouth and restore hydration.

To use in tea, place one teaspoon of the powder in a glass of steaming tea and stir. The powder will dissolve in the hot liquid.

For psoriasis and dry skin, mix one teaspoon of powder with one tablespoon of unscented petroleum jelly and spread on the dry skin. For maximum benefit and to prevent the petroleum jelly from getting on your clothes, cover the area with a sterile gauze for at least three hours or overnight.

Planting and Growing Bishop's Weed

Bishop's Weed grows between one and two feet tall with a maximum width of four feet. It grows extremely well in all climates and once planted, does not need maintained or replanted. The same plants will continue growing year after year. The white flowers bloom in the early summer and tower above the rest of the plant.

Bishop's Weed is a very common adornment at nursing homes and for anyone who does not wish to do a lot of maintenance in their flower garden. It rarely needs pruned and will not become overgrown with weeds.

It is also worth noting that Bishop's Weed is a weed. Therefore, it is recommended that gardeners who wish to grow Bishop's weed do so in an area where it can easily be contained. Sidewalks, flower bed edging, bricks, stones, and well-maintained grass are all considered barriers against the unwanted spreading of the plant.

Bishop's weed can be grown in any soil type, with any amount of sunlight and watering. To grow Bishop's Weed, buy one or more plants from your local nursery or home gardening centre. Dig a bed as if you were planting flowers. Make sure there is a natural barrier between the Bishop's Weed bed and the other plants in your yard. The only exception is Hosta. Hosta's can be planted alongside Bishop Weed because they are resilient enough to hold their own ground and will not be overtaken.

Plant the Bishop's weed root deep and cover with soil. After planting, water the plants lightly to help them set. They will not need any further care after the initial watering.

Warnings

Bishop's Weed does not have any known allergies or side effects.

3. Brier Hip

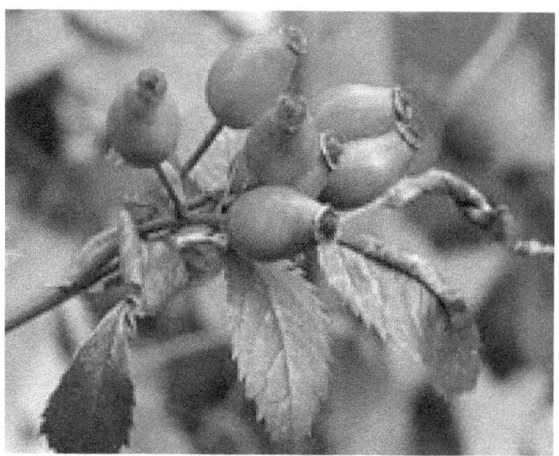

Origins

Brier Hip is also known as Witches Brier and Rose Hip. It was discovered centuries ago in India and written about by Gaius Plinius Secundus in his medical texts. Brier Hip is a shrub that grows between three and 16 feet tall and contains small, red, berry-like fruits and white or pink flowers. The leaves and stems contain prickly hooked spines, which allow it to grow up trees and trellises. The fruit is edible and has a slightly acidic, sweet taste. It is very popular in Sweden and Italy, where it is used to flavour foods and drinks.

Ailments

Brier Hip is used to treat bladder and kidney irritation and diarrhoea. It is well-known for its astringent and diuretic properties and is most often brewed into a tea and/or made into preserves, syrup, and jelly. The scent is often used to relieve anxiety, depression, and stress, and to promote total body relaxation.

How It's Used

Brier hip is typically consumed as a tea for urinary and kidney ailments, and it can be made into preserves and jellies for consumption on toast and bread. It is recommended that individuals treating bladder and kidney ailments drink three cups of a tea per day. The preserves and jellies are not as effective because of the high sugar content.

Recipes

Brier Hip Preserves

4 Cups Fresh Brier Hip Fruits
3 Cups White Sugar Or Your favourite Sugar Alternative
2 Cups Cold Water
4 Tablespoons Lemon Juice
1 Large Pot
1 Long Handled Wooden Spoon
2 16 Ounce Mason Jars With Lids
1 Stove Top Porcelain Canner

Cut and remove the stems and seeds from the fruit. This is best done by slicing open the fruit and removing the seeds by hand. You can throw away the seeds or save them for planting. Combine the water and sugar in your pot and turn the flame on high. Stir the mixture until the sugar is dissolved in the water. Add the seeded rose hips and lemon juice to the sugar water solution. Continue to cook until the rose hips are soft and the mixture is thick and red.

To safely store the preserves, you'll need a canning kit and two, 16 ounce jars. Follow the directions on your canner to safely sterilize and store the preserves. Once canned, the preserves will last for years.

Brier Hip Tea

2 Tablespoons Dried and Crushed Brier Hips
3 Cups White Sugar Or Your favourite Sugar Alternative
2 1/4 Cups Cold Water

Pour the water into the pan and bring it to a boil. After the water is at a rolling boil, add the dried brier hips and boil for 10 minutes. Turn off the heat and strain the water into a tea glass. If the flavour is too bitter, honey or sugar can be added.

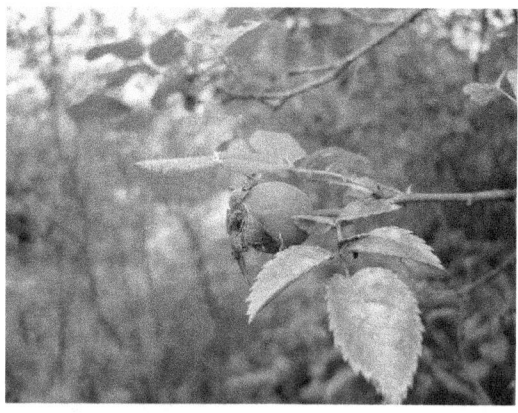

Brier Hip grows well in all climates. To ready the seeds for planting, pour eight ounces of water in a 16 ounce jar and add one teaspoon of bleach. Drop the seeds into the jar and seal with the lid. Shake the jar vigorously to mix the seeds, water, and bleach. Set the jar on the counter and wait 30 minutes. The majority of the seeds should settle at the bottom of the jar. If there are seeds floating in the water, remove them. They will not grow.

Drain the rest of the water off the seeds and lay the seeds in a single layer on a double-thick line of paper towel. Allow the seeds to dry overnight. In the morning, plant the seeds in your flower bed. Plant the seeds in fertile, well-draining soil with partial sun, water directly after planting. Brier Hips do not need watered unless there is no rain forecast for an extended amount of time. It is recommended to plant the seeds near a healthy tree or a trellis. Brier Hips do best when they have something to climb, and this prevents the fruit from lying on the ground and rotting on the stem.

Warnings

There are no side effects associated with eating Brier Hips. However, if you are worried about an allergic reaction, test by drinking a small cup of tea. If no reaction or rash develops, you are not allergic to the plant.

4. Coal Tar

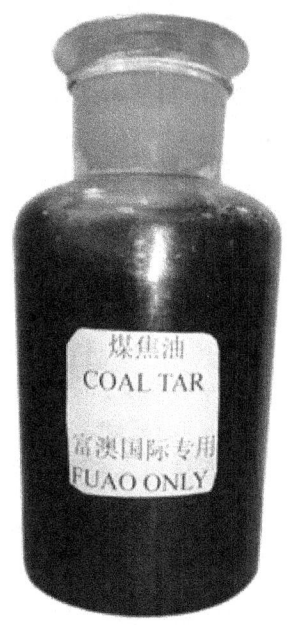

Origins

Coal tar is a by-product of distilling coal and wood with heat and has been around since the late 1850s. Coal tar was first used by farmers and the Amish to treat skin wounds and rashes and to remove splinters and foreign object from the skin. It can also be used to treat moderate and severe coughs, vomiting, diarrhoea, and tuberculosis. In fact, early doctors used coal tar as a prescribed treatment for the symptoms of tuberculosis.

There are two types of coal tar, including low temperature coal tar and high temperature coal tar. High temperature coal tar is created when the coal and/or wood is heated between 1,650 degrees Fahrenheit to 2,200 degrees Fahrenheit.

Coal tar is also known as creosote, and most people are familiar with it from wood burning fireplaces or coal burning stoves. It is the soot left in the bottom of the fireplace or wood burning stove. However, the ashes and soot in fireplaces and wood burning stoves should not be used as a herbal remedy. Many commercial coals and firewood have been treated with chemicals.

Ailments

Coal tar is used to treat a wide range of skin ailments, including psoriasis, severe dry skin, red scaly lesions, and eczema. The exact reasons why coal tar works are unknown, but it seems to work like an antiseptic and a moisturiser.

How It's Used

Coal tar can be found in shampoos, ointments, soaps, and as a poultice. It is used topically to treat a wide range of skin ailments from dry skin and minor cuts to psoriasis and eczema. The products can contain anywhere from one per cent to 20 per cent coal tar.

Some coal tar remedies require a prescription from a licensed doctor. Others can be bought over the counter. Creams and ointments should be applied to problems areas on the skin. The soaps can be used to wash the entire body, and shampoos should be used on the hair and scalp.

Products

Cream
Shampoo
Ointment
Bar Soap

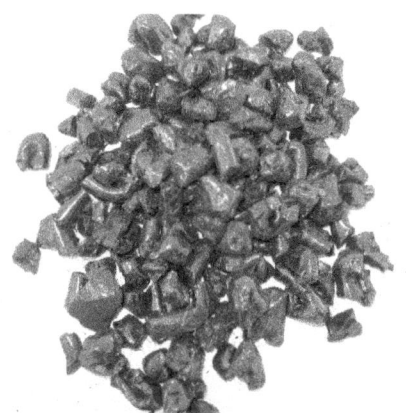

Finding Coal Tar for Remedies

Coal Tar, by itself, cannot readily be purchased. The only types of coal tar available commercially are for paving roads and sealing roofs. This is not the same coal tar used in herbal remedies. However, you can make your own coal tar treatments by using activated charcoal, which can be purchased in pill form from any well-stocked vitamin shop. To get the charcoal, simply break open the pill and pour the contents into a small bowl.

Black Tar Drawing Salve

Black Tar Drawing Salve is a popular Amish recipe for removing foreign object from the skin and treating minor skin wounds and infections.

Ingredients

2 Tablespoons Vitamin E Oil (Can be purchased at any health food store for about $7. Just make sure it's 100% Vitamin E Oil.)
2 Tablespoons High-Quality Virgin Olive Oil (Do not buy the cheap options.They may not be 100% virgin olive oil. Many inexpensive olive oils are cut with vegetable oil, which reduces its effectiveness.)
2 Tablespoons Amish Honey (Can be purchased at any Amish farmers market or in health food stores.)
2 Tablespoons Coconut Oil (Can be Purchased At Most Grocers)
4 Tablespoons Pure, Unscented Beeswax (Can be purchased at any vitamin store)
4 Tablespoons Activated Charcoal Powder (Can be purchased in caplets at any vitamin store. Just make sure it's caplets and not pills. Break open the caplets to retrieve the char coal powder)
6 Tablespoons Bentonite Or Rhassoul Clay (Can be purchased online, in spice stores, and in vitamin stores. Make sure it is 100% organic and contains no fillers.)

Supplies

Make sure you only use supplies and equipment you will not need for anything else. Once you make a herbal remedy with your pots, pans, spoons, and measuring cups, those items cannot be used for anything else.

1 Wooden Spoon
1 Food Thermometer
1 Medium Sized Stainless Steel or Iron Saucepan
1 16 Ounce Canning jar Or large Medicinal Jar With A Tight-Fitting Lid

Pour all of the ingredients into the pan except the activated char coal and turn the stove on to medium heat. Stir all of the ingredients until the beeswax is completely melted and all of the oils are combined. Heat the mixture to 180 degrees Fahrenheit for between 15 and 20 minutes. Use the thermometer to gauge the temperature and keep it steady for the allotted time. Do not walk away from the mixture and do not add the activated charcoal.

After the allotted time has passed, turn off the burner and move the pan to a cold burner. Add the activated charcoal and stir until it is thoroughly combined. This should turn the colour from the mixture from yellow/tan to black. It should also cause the mixture to thicken slightly.

Let the mixture cool to room temperature. It will become thicker as it cools. Afterward, put the concoction into the glass jar and seal tightly. It will last up to two years in a location that is below 72 degrees and free of sunlight.

To use for cuts and object removal, put a little of the mixture over the cut, splinter, or foreign object in the skin and cover with a large band-aide or gauze. For embedded objects, it may take two or three days for the object to fully come out of the skin. The gauze or band-aide should be changed daily. This is best done after a shower and after the skin has completely dried. If you are allergic to gauze or bandages, take two Benadryl after application and it will reduce the allergic reaction to the glue in the adhesive bandage.

To use over eczema and skin lesions caused by psoriasis, apply a little of the salve on the dry patches or skin lesions and cover with a gauze bandage. The bandage prevents the coal tar salve from getting on your clothing and staining it. The bandage should be left on for several hours or overnight.

Warnings

Coal tar can stain skin, clothing, and hair, and make users more susceptible to sunburns. Individuals should test a small section of their skin for allergies before using coal tar regularly. Coal tar also considered a carcinogen. Though, coal tar has only been known to cause cancer in miners and other individuals who are around coal and creosote on a daily basis and over the course of many years. Coal tar and creosote can cause prostate and testicular cancer and diminish lung function.

5. Daisies (Bellis Perennis)

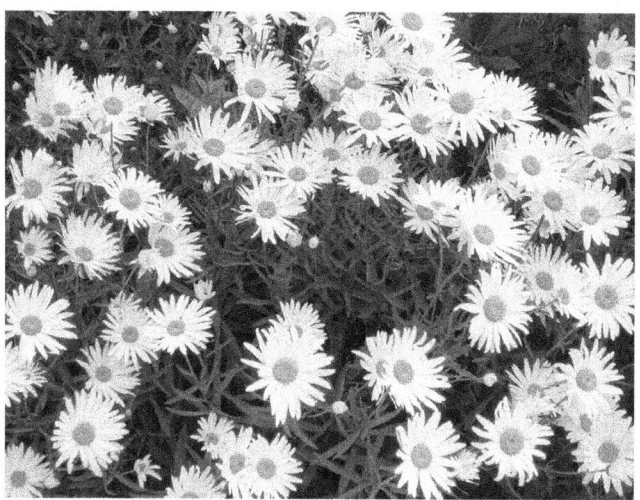

Origins

Daises were first used in herbal medicine in the 1500s by the Europeans. They brewed the leaves, stems, and roots of the plant into teas, and used the flower petals and leaves in solutions of warm water to cleanse wounds.

Today, we know about daisies from flower and botanical gardens as they are highly prized for the beauty of their flowers. However, they can still be used as medicine and are quite effective at treating a wide range of conditions.

Ailments

Daisies can be used to treat problems associated with heavy menstruation and severe headaches, including migraines. The flowers can also help heal ulcers, dry up excess mucus, and reduce inflammation of the mucus membranes. Daisy ointments and poultices can be applied topically to relieve arthritis and bruising. Women who have just given birth may use daisy water to cleanse the area between their vagina and anus. This area typically tears during a vaginal birth, and the daisy water is said to aide in healing and prevents infection. Chewing the leaves can aide in healing wounds and ulcers inside the mouth.

How It's Used

The leaves, flowers, and roots can be brewed into a tea or washed and placed in warm water for cleansing the body. The plant contains clotting properties and astringent properties, which can be used to close and heal wounds.

Recipes

Daisy water

Ingredients

5 or 6 Fresh Leaves
16 Ounces Of Water

Run the hot water on your tap until the water is steaming. Collect 16 ounces and pour it into a bowl.

Add the leaves and stir. Let it sit for 10 minutes. Dip a clean wash cloth in the water and cleanse the desired areas. This should help in healing minor cuts and wounds on the skin and injuries sustained while delivering a baby.

Daisy Tea

Ingredients

2 Tablespoons of fresh or dried leaves
16 Ounces Of Water

Boil 16 ounces of water on the stove. Once the water is at a rolling boil, add the leaves and turn off the burner. Let the leaves and water steep for between 5 and 10 minutes. The longer it steeps, the stronger the tea.

Strain the leaves and pour into a glass. The tea can be drunk up to three times a day.

Leaves for Chewing

Ingredients

2 or 3 Fresh Leaves From The Daisy Plant

Two or three fresh daisy leaves should be rinsed thoroughly with cold water to remove any dirt or debris from the leaves. Once the leaves are clean, chew them for 15 to 20 minutes. This should aide in the healing of any mouth sores or ulcers.

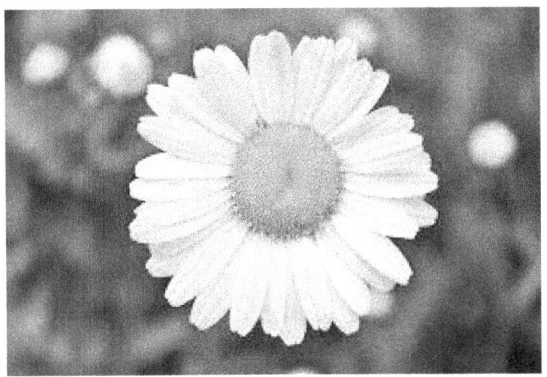

Growing Daisies

Daisy seeds can be procured from any nursery or home improvement store. Plant the seeds about half an inch in loose soil and water lightly. The seedlings will take between one and two weeks to sprout. The flowers will bloom in the summer after the plant has matured. Daisies can be grown in any climate. They can even be grown indoors in flower pots.

Warnings

Individuals who are allergic to daisies should not use any remedies concocted from the plant. Allergy symptoms include rashes, breathing problems, hives, and excess mucus. Pregnant and lactating women should avoid using the plant as a herbal remedy and anyone with blood clots should not use any part of the daisy for consumption.

6. Figwort (Scrophularia Nodosa)

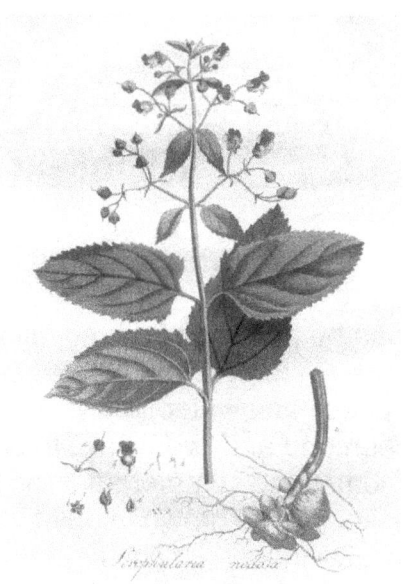

Scrophularia nodosa

Origins

Figwort was first discovered centuries ago in Europe and North America and was used to treat tuberculosis, haemorrhoids and throat inflammation and irritation. It was ground into poultices and used to treat dry skin, eczema and psoriasis. It was also used in Asian medicine to heal burns, promote whole body health and to heal draining and oozing infected sores and boils.

Today, figwort is used to detox the body and promote balance and good health.

The plant can be identified by its small greenish-brown flowers and pill like seeds. The leaves are oval and pointed at the end and contain spine-like protrusions along the outer edge of the leaves. They can be found in the cooler climates of North America, Europe and Asia, during the summer months.

Ailments

Figwort can be used to detox the body, sooth throat inflammation and irritation and to aide in healing dry skin caused by eczema and psoriasis. As a tincture or ointment, it can be put on and inside large, pussy, infected wounds and boils to promote healing.

How It's Used

Figwort is most commonly brewed into a tea and crushed into poultices and ointments. It is safe to put on skin and to eat. Some countries even use it as a vegetable, and it was rumoured to feed the Germans during WWII and prevent hundreds of families from starving to death.

Recipes

Figwort Tea

Ingredients

16 Ounces Water

2 Tablespoons Fresh Or Dried Leaves

Boil the water in a pan. Once the water is boiling, add the dried or fresh leaves. Turn off the heat and let the mixture steep for between 10 and 15 minutes. The longer it steeps, the more potent the tea. Strain the leaves from the water and pour into a glass. This should be drunk three times a day. The tea will taste bitter, and some people find it unpalatable. If the tea is too bitter, add a little honey and/or lemon. This will neutralize the bitter taste and add a hint sweetness.

Figwort Oil

Figwort oil is used in the making of ointments and creams.

Ingredients

1 Cup Fresh Figwort Leaves and Flowers
8 Ounces Carrier Oil (Olive Oil, Avocado Oil, Sesame Seed Oil, Rose Hip Oil)
1 16 Ounce Mason jar
1 Glass Oil Bottle with Spout

Place the leaves in the jar and cover with your choice of carrier oil. It's best to cover the leaves until the oil is about 1/2 inch to 1 inch above the leaves. Seal the jar with the lid and shake well. Set aside in your cabinet or pantry. Shake the bottle once a day for at least 14 days. This can be performed for up to 45 days. At the end of your desired time-frame, strain the leaves from the oil and place the herb infused oil in a separate clean jar with a lid. It is now ready for your other recipes, or it can be used as is as a massage oil and for aromatherapy.

Figwort Ointment

Ingredients

1/4 Cup Beeswax or Unscented Petroleum Jelly
3/4 Cup Figwort Oil

Place the beeswax or petroleum jelly in a small pan that you do not intend to use for anything else. Once you use a pan for a herbal remedy, it can never be used for food preparation or cooking again.

On low heat, stir the base until it is completely melted. Add the figwort oil and stir until it is completely combined with your base. Turn off the heat and pour the contents into an air tight, glass jar. Seal with a lid and store in a pantry or cabinet.

Once it cools, it can be used on dry skin, eczema, psoriasis, boils, and infected wounds. For added disinfectant properties, one to two tablespoons of pure Amish honey can be added to the mixture while it is boiling in the pan.

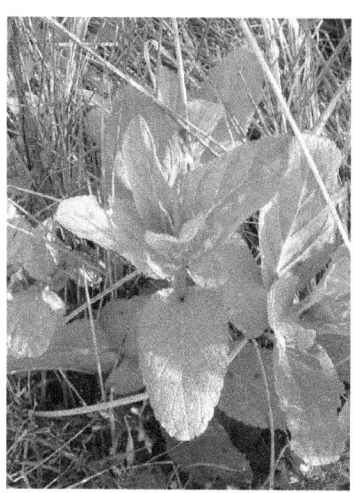

Figwort Tincture

Ingredients

1 Cup of Fresh or Dried Figwort Leaves and Flowers
12 Ounces Clear, 95 proof Vodka
16 Ounce Mason jar
1 Tincture Bottle with Eyedropper Lid

Place the fresh or dried leaves into the tincture jar and cover them with the Vodka. You want the Vodka to completely cover all of the leaves. This is best done by filling the jar 1/2 inch to one inch above the leaves. Seal the jar with the lid and place it in a cool, dry and dark area. Let it sit for at least two weeks.

After two weeks, strain the leaves from the alcohol and pour the alcohol into a tincture bottle with an eyedropper lid. To use, simply put two or three drops into your mouth or your morning tea or coffee.

Growing Figwort

Figwort can be grown from a seed and thrives well in almost all climates. It should be planted in shady areas and watered well. It does not like dry conditions. Most individuals choose to grow their figwort plants in planter boxes with very few drainage holes.

Warnings

Pregnant women should not use this herb. It may cause birth defects and deformities in the foetus.

7. Garden/ Lemon Balm (Melissa Officinalis)

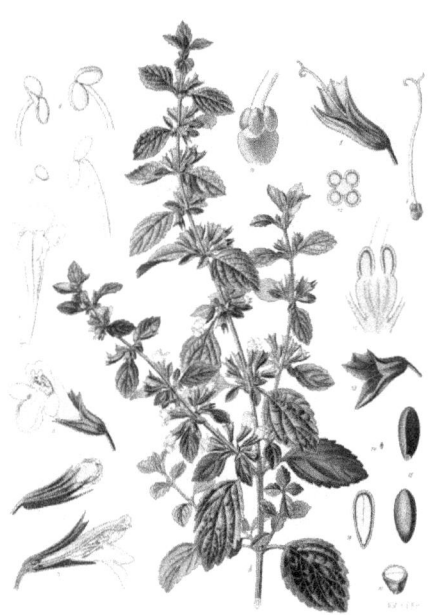

Origins

Lemon Balm was first discovered in the Mediterranean more than 2,000 years ago by the Romans and used to help heal infected cuts and scrapes. It was consumed by pregnant women to help alleviate morning sickness, and it was drunk as a tea and used as a tincture to relieve toothaches and gum soreness.

The plant is characterized by bright to deep green leaves that are scalloped and pointed. Its flowers are typically white or yellow contain a slight lemon scent. They grow between 18 inches to two feet tall and 18 to three feet wide. The flowers bloom in the early summer.

Ailments

Lemon Balm is used to treat a wide variety of ailments, including anxiety, depression and stress, and it can even be sprayed on the skin and used as a mosquito repellent. It contains antibacterial, antioxidant and antiviral properties and has been shown to treat herpes when taken as a tea.

There is some research that suggests in helps Alzheimer's patients because it helps stabilize moods and enhances cognitive performance on basic Alzheimer's tests. It may also help individuals with Graves' disease and Hyperthyroidism due to its ability to stunt the hormone thyrotropin.

How It's Used

The leaves and flowers of the Lemon Balm plant can be eaten raw or cooked and added to salads. It can also be used as an essential oil and tincture, and it can be brewed into a tea. The leaves and flowers are highly prized for their lemon scent, which calms nerves and promotes relaxation.

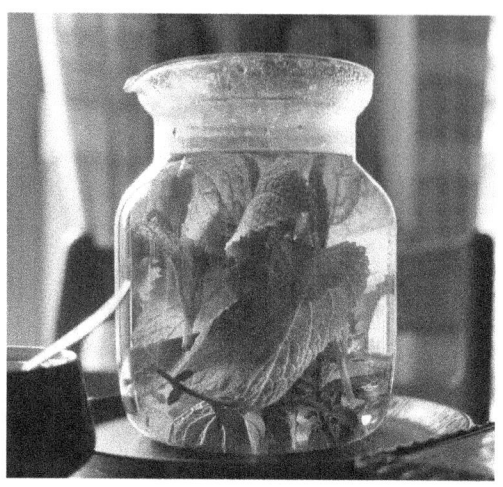

Lemon Balm Tea

2 To 3 Tablespoons Dried or fresh leaves and/or
Flowers
16 Ounces Of water

Boil the water on the stove and add the leaves after
the water reaches a rolling boil. Turn off the heat and
let the leaves steep for between five and 10 minutes.
After words, strain the leaves from the water, and pour
the water into a glass. The tea should have a pleasant
lemon smell and taste. Honey or another sweetener
can be added to the tea to increase its sweetness.
This can be consumed up to three times a day.

Lemon Balm Oil

8 Ounces of Carrier Oil
1 Cup or Dried or Fresh Leaves and Flowers
16 Ounce Mason jar

1 Oil Jar with Spout

Put the leaves in the 16 ounce mason jar and cover completely with the carrier oil. Screw the lid on tightly and set in a cool, dark place. Leave the mixture sit for at least two weeks, but no more than six weeks. After words, strain the leaves from the oil using a fine mesh strainer, cheesecloth or coffee filter and funnel. Pour the infused oil into an oil bottle. It is now ready to use as a massage oil, for dipping bread and over salads or in other recipes. It can also be used as an aromatic massage oil to relax the mind and body.

Lemon Balm Tincture

1 Cup of Fresh Dried Leaves
1 Bottle of 95 proof Vodka
16 Ounce Mason jar

Put the leaves in the mason jar and cover them completely with the vodka. Seal the jar with the lid and store untouched for at least two weeks. After words, strain the liquid into a tincture bottle and cap it with an eyedropper lid. The tincture should be dripped onto the tongue or added to tea and coffee.

Lemon Balm as A Food

The leaves of the Lemon Balm plant can be added to salads and sandwiches or cooked as a vegetable in butter or water. It is safe to consume the leaves in any quantity.

Growing Lemon Balm

Lemon Balm makes a great addition to any garden and will grow well in most climates. It's easy to grow and prefers partial sun and damp soil. It's best to plant it in an area where it will receive either morning sun or evening sun, but not both. It thrives in well-draining soil and does not need watering unless there is no rain in the weather forecast.

Warnings

There are no adverse effects from ingesting or using Lemon Balm.

8. Hibiscus

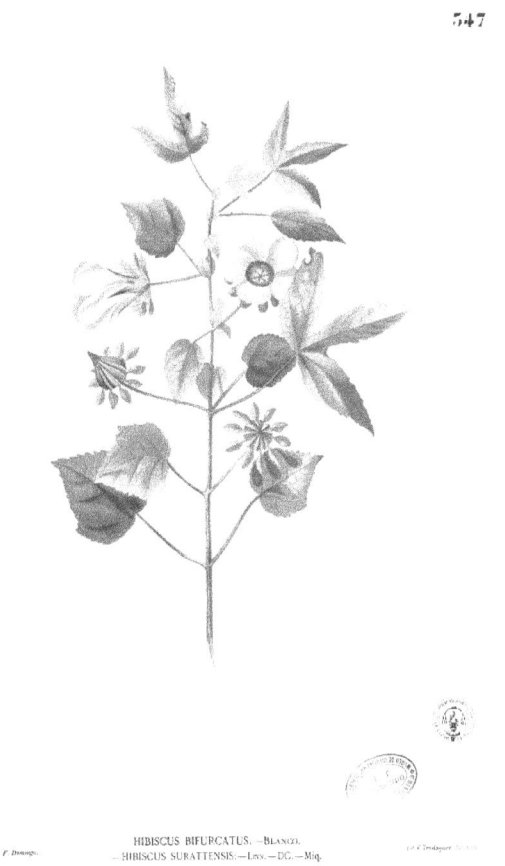

HIBISCUS BIFURCATUS. —BLANCO.
HIBISCUS SUBATTENSIS. —Lixx.—DC.—Miq.

Origins

Hibiscus originated in Asia and is one of the many herbs and plants associated with traditional Chinese medicine. The name Hibiscus incorporates more than

200 different varieties of the plant, and all of the varieties can be used for tea and as a herbal remedy. The tea can be consumed either hot or cold, and it can be mixed with other spices for a more potent effect. In some Asian countries, it is mixed with wine to add flavour and increase the antioxidant properties of the wine and Hibiscus.

Ailments

Drinking hibiscus tea can lower blood pressure and bad cholesterol, improve metabolism and heal respiratory and lung infections due to its high vitamin C content and antioxidant properties. It can be used to relieve bladder and kidney infections and lessen severe coughs and to treat stomach and intestinal problems.

In some studies, it has been shown to reduce tumours associated with cancer and can enhance conventional cancer treatments. Individuals with cancer should speak with their doctor about drinking Hibiscus tea along with their treatments. This is to prevent the possibility of receiving too much treatment.

How It's Used

Hibiscus is most often brewed into a tea and consumed. The calyx of the plant produces a rich red tea that is pleasing to the palette. For added health benefits, fresh lemon juice or Amish honey can be added to the tea. Lemon and honey are both power antibacterial and contain antioxidant properties, and they will enhance the effects of the tea.

Harvesting

The best part of the plant to use for tea is the calyx. This can be found covering the flowers that have not yet bloomed or under the flowers once they have bloomed. These leaves should be gently broken away from the plant, washed and dried before use. In the event that you cannot find the leaves, the leaves and flowers of the plant can also be brewed into a tea, but the tea will not be as aromatic or strong.

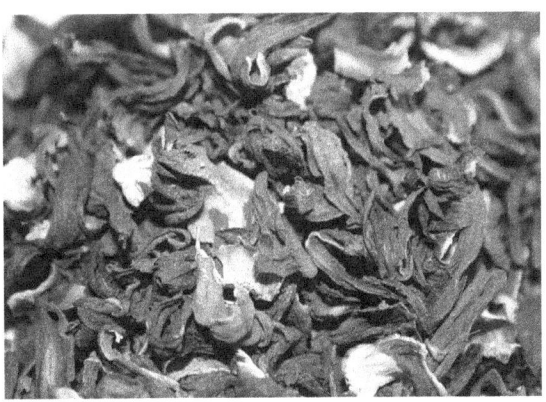

Drying Hibiscus Leaves

Wash the leaves thoroughly under cold water to remove any dirt, debris and bugs. Dry them gently with a paper towel and lay them across a wire rack. Make sure the air can reach the leaves on both sides. If the air cannot reach both sides of the leaves, you risk the leaves molding. If the leaves mold, throw them away. They cannot be consumed.

Let the leaves sit undisturbed on the wire rack for two

weeks. After words, crush them and put them in an air-tight glass jar. They should stay fresh for up to 12 months.

Recipes

Hibiscus Tea

Ingredients

2 Tablespoons Dried Leaves
16 Ounces Water

Boil the water on the stove. Once it reaches a rolling boil, drop the leaves into the water and give it a good stir. Turn off the heat and let the tea steep for five minutes. The water should turn red. Strain the leaves from the water and pour into a glass. Hibiscus tea can be sweetened with honey or sugar and flavored with lemon or vanilla. This can be consumed up to three times a day for the duration of the illness or for weight loss.

For overall general health benefits and to lower blood pressure and cholesterol, consume 16 ounces of tea once a day. This is best done in the morning as the plant is a natural diuretic.

Growing Hibiscus

Hibiscus prefers partial to full sun and grows between four and 10 feet tall. Its flowers are pink, red, and red-orange with a single long stigma, and it has green, pointed leaves. It thrives well in moderate to warm temperatures and can be planted in areas that have four seasons. It is favoured by gardeners because of its ability to attract butterflies.

The hibiscus can be bought as a seedling or a plant and transplanted, or it can be grown from seeds. It is very easy to manage and can thrive in a wide variety of soil conditions. It only needs watered if the soil is extremely dry.

Warnings

Hibiscus has blood pressure lowering qualities and should not be consumed by individuals that already have low blood pressure or by people on birth control or with hormone issues. It is also recommended that individuals first consume the tea at home on their days off. It has been known to cause impairment similar to alcohol in some individuals, and in extreme cases it can cause hallucinations. Building up a tolerance to the tea can lessen its negative effects. However, if a severe reaction occurs, discontinue using Hibiscus.

9. Oil Pulling

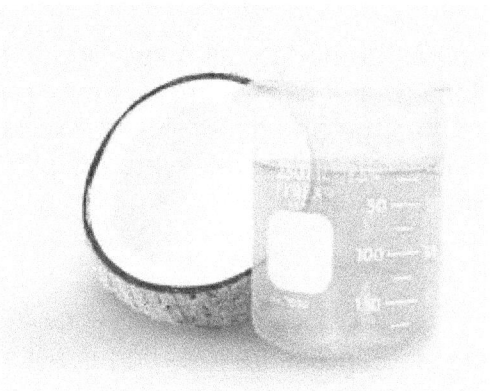

Origins

Something my Grandma swears by, a ritual she does every day, normally with Olive or Coconut Oil is oil pulling. Some may say oil pulling is an old wives tale, and they could be right - saying that though, she does seem to be pretty fit for her age (which she won't let me publish) and her teeth are in excellent order.

Oil pulling has been around for centuries and involves swishing sesame seed or coconut oil around in the mouth as if it were mouthwash. It was first developed in India and recommended in Indian Ayurvedic texts, which are alternative medical texts.

These texts describe using oil pulling to heal and alleviate a multitude of ailments, including receding gums and cavities, and the people in India have been using oil pulling since before there were formal studies on its benefits. Oil pulling aides in oral health and it is said that individuals who oil pull will never have cavities or infected gums or oral health problems. Some people even report being able to grow back gums and tooth enamel through the use of oil pulling. It is also said to balance the body and promote weigh loss in overweight people.

Ailments

Oil pulling has been used to increase oral health for centuries. It is said to heal and prevent gum disease and tooth decay, and it can even detox the liver and the body and aide is weight loss. In short, it helps balance the body and remove harmful toxins so the body can focus on fighting legitimate bacterial and viral threats.

How It's Used

Choose your favourite 100% oil, including coconut oil, sesame seed oil, or sunflower oil. Keep the bottle in your bathroom just like you would regular mouthwash. Right after you get out of bed, put one tablespoon of oil in your mouth and swish it around and through your teeth. Make sure to get every part of your mouth with the oil. Do not gargle the oil. You do not want it sliding down your throat.

Use your cell phone timer and set it for 20 minutes. Continuously swish the oil around in your mouth for the entire 20 minutes. This should be done before you eat or drink anything or brush your teeth. The goal of this treatment is to pull all the toxins out of your body through the mucus membranes in your mouth. It also promotes the secretion of saliva, which is said to have health benefits.

If you cannot swish for the entire 20 minutes, try ten minutes at a time for a total of 20 minutes. You can rinse your mouth out with water in between sessions, but do not drink any water. For maximum benefit, this should be performed on a daily basis. Most people report health benefits after one month of use.

Warnings

There are no side effects to oil pulling. It is 100% natural. However, some individuals may experience headaches and upset stomach. This is due to the removal of toxins from the body and should go away after a few days.

10. Pine Tar

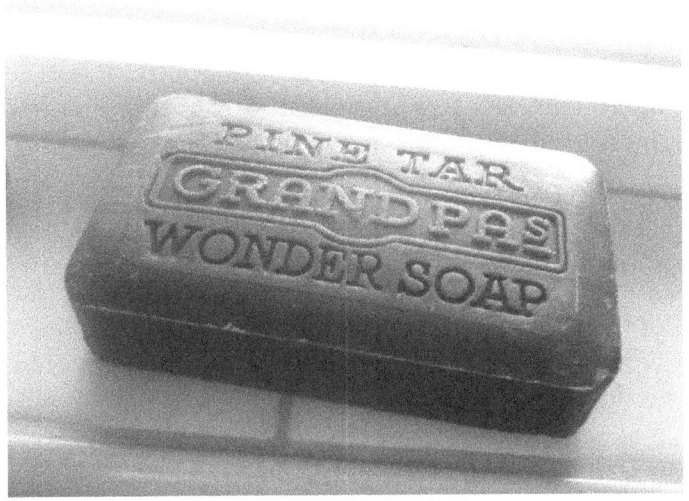

Origins

Pine tar has been around for centuries. It was first used to waterproof and preserve the wood of sailing ships. Pine tar is created by burning pine wood at very hot temperatures, which is exactly the way coal tar is produced, and pine tar is used for exactly the same remedies as pine tar, except pine tar has been noted to help with moderate to severe coughs from viral and bacterial infections.

Pine tar cough medicine was very popular in America from the 1860s until the 1960s, and it was sold in almost every pharmacy. It only lost its appeal after more modern cough medicines came on the market, such as Nyquil and Alka-Seltzer.

Ailments

Pine tar can be used to relieve dry skin, itching and flaking, dandruff, rashes and allergic reactions from poison ivy and oak, psoriasis, and eczema. It can be combined with several other ingredients to help ease coughs and promote the expulsion of mucus.

Pine Tar Extraction

Pine tar is easily extracted at home using a large cast iron pot with a lid, yellow pine wood chips, a long yellow pine board and enough coal or other wood to start a fire.

Place a row of pine chips tightly in the bottom of the cast iron pot and put the lid on the pot. Put a pile of clay under the pot. Sink the pot upside down in the clay. If the clay does not cover the lid, add more clay. This is to keep the pot stable while you build and burn a fire to extract the tar.

Take the longer yellow pine board and cut several grooves in it. The pine tar will congeal in the grooves and slide down the board into a waiting pot.

Put the low end of the board in another clean pot or small bucket. Create a pile of concrete blocks that's taller than the cast iron pot and rest the board on the blocks. Make sure the cast iron pot is located near the high side of the board and under the board. The heat from the fire needs to reach the board. However, do not build the fire so big that the flames touch the board. The goal is not to light the board on fire, but to heat it to a point where the sap drips down the board and into the pot.

Now, start a small fire on top of the cast iron pot with untreated wood and/or coal. It is very important that the wood and/or coal does not contain any added chemicals. If they do, those chemicals could get into your pine tar and reduce its effectiveness and even cause allergic reactions.

Make sure the fire burns continuously for at least 30 minutes. It will take that long for the board to heat up and start to make the pine tar. Do not walk away from the fire once it is burning.

You can put out the fire after the tar starts flowing down the board. This should yield at least two cups of pine tar.

How It's Used

Pine tar can be mixed with honey and beeswax to form a salve that can be placed on cuts, scrapes, dry skin, and skin lesions. It can be mixed with shampoo for dandruff, and it can be made into bar soap for hand washing and showers. If you are mixing your own pine tar into your shampoo and soap bottles, make sure the pine tar is not more than 25% of the mixture.

Recipes

Pine Tar Salve

To make pine tar salve, simply follow the recipe for coal tar salve and substitute pine tar for the coal tar. This salve can be used exactly as you would use coal tar salve. It should be stored in a collared glass jar with a lid to prevent light degradation.

Pine Tar Soap

Pine tar soap is great for relieving dry skin and lesions associated with eczema and psoriasis.

Ingredients

All equipment, pots, pans and spoons used to make soap cannot be used for any other purpose. Store them in a safe location away from your kitchen so no one accidentally uses them. Once you use cooking equipment and utensils to make soap, it cannot be used for anything else. Most people prefer to store the items in their utility rooms.

1 Large Cast Iron or Stainless Steel Pot
1 Large Plastic or Wooden Spoon
1 Roll of Wax Paper
Small Boxes or Something to Use as a Soap Mold
1 Bar Of Soap Base (32 Ounces)
2 to 8 Ounces of Pine Tar (No more than 25 per cent of the total mixture)
Your Choice Of Essential Oils

Turn the burner on and place the soap base in the pot. The soap should start to melt almost immediately. With your wooden spoon, stir the soap as it melts. Once it is completely melted, add the pine tar and a few drops of essential oil. Stir the mixture until it is completely combined.

If you prefer, you can also add coconut oil and/or beeswax for extra moisturizing.

Once everything is completely melted and combined, turn off the heat. Line your soap mold with the wax paper. Pour the hot soap into the mold and cover with another piece of wax paper. Allow the soap to completely cool for at least eight hours. As the soap cools, it will harden into a bar.

Once the soap is cool, remove it from the mold and pull off the wax paper. It is now ready to use.

This recipe is perfect for individuals who have never made soap because it does not contain any harsh or toxic chemicals.

Other Soap Recipes

Pine tar can be added to almost any soap recipe. If you're familiar with making soap, simply follow the directions for your favourite soap and add no more than 25% pine tar as compared to the entire recipe. More than 25% pine tar can make the soap too harsh to use and cause dry skin instead of healing it.

Warnings

Very few people are allergic to pine tar, but if you think you might be, test the pine tar on a small section of skin. If a rash or redness appears, discontinue use. If you decide to use a soap recipe with lye, remember to wear protective gloves and eyewear. Lye is very acidic in its pure form. The acidity is neutralized during the soap making process.

11. Roses and Rose Petals

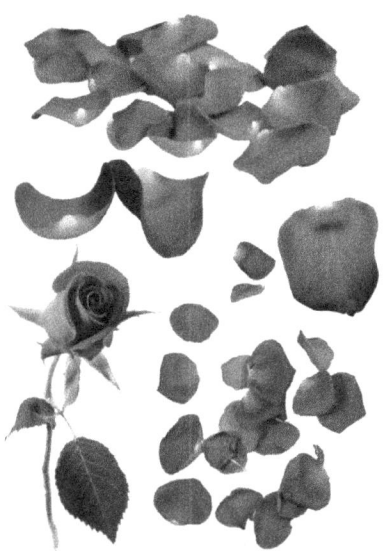

Origins

Roses have been around for more than 70 million years, and used for their medicinal purposes since before the birth of Christ. Ancient humans would bath in rose water and drink rose tea. They are one of the oldest plants known to man and were first discovered and used by the ancient Romans for decoration and medicine. The Chinese, Romans and the Egyptians were the first to choose roses by their specific color, and images of roses can be found carved into ancient tombs and on tablets and statues.

Today, roses are better known for their fragrance and their association with love, romance and well-wishes, but they can still be used as a herbal remedy.

Ailments

Rose petals can alleviate constipation, aide in digestion, ease headaches and pain associated with PMS, and cramping from menstruation. The petals are also very high in vitamin C and can increase the body's immune system to heal bacterial infections and colds and the flu. Bathing and washing in rose petal water can help heal skin infections and relieve dry skin. Using a rose petal mouthwash can help freshen breath and heal mouth sores.

How It's Used

Rose petals can be put directly into warm bath water for a refreshing and relaxing bath. They can be brewed into tea to aide with digestive problems, diarrhoea, and menstrual cramps. When they are infused with vinegar, they form a refreshing and detoxifying mouthwash, and rose oil can be used for its aromatic properties and as a massage oil.

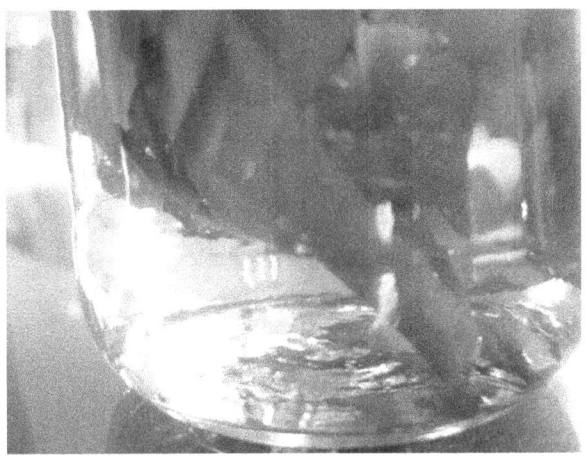

Rose Water

Ingredients

3 Cups Freshly Washed Rose Petals
Water
Ice
Large Pot with a Glass Lid
16 Ounce Mason jar

Place the 16 ounce mason jar in the center of the pot. Surround the jar with lots of water and add the rose petals. Make sure no water or rose petals get inside your mason jar. This is where the rose water will collect.

Turn the burner on high and place the lid upside down in the pot. The steam from the water will rise, collect on the lid, flow down the sloping edge and drip into the mason jar. To accelerate the process, you can put six to eight ice cubes on top of the lid. This will help the steam condense faster. Stop the process when the jar is 3/4 full of rose water. Any further collecting will result in a diluted product.

This can be used to clean wounds and to treat eczema and psoriasis.

Rose Vinegar Mouthwash

1/2 Cup Freshly Washed Rose Petals
16 Ounces Apple Cider or Red Wine Vinegar (Do not use white or balsamic vinegar)
1 Jug Distilled Water

Place the washed and dried rose petals in the mason jar and cover completely with vinegar. Seal the jar with a lid and place it in a cool, dark area. Let the mixture sit for between one and two weeks. Once the allotted time has passed, strain the rose petals from the vinegar and place it in another glass jar. To use, get a glass and add 1/2 cup distilled water. Place two tablespoons of the rose vinegar in the water and use just as you would use store-bought mouthwash. This will clean and disinfect your mouth and gums.

Rose Tea

1 To 2 Tablespoons Dried and Crushed Rose Petals
16 Ounces Water

Boil the water and add the dried rose petals. Turn off the heat and allow the mixture steep for five minutes. The tea should be very fragrant. Strain the petals from the water, and pour into a tea cup. For a sweeter flavour, add one teaspoon organic or Amish honey.

Rose Massage Oil

2 Cups washed and dried rose petals
16 Ounces Carrier Oil

Place the rose petals in the mason jar and cover them with the carrier oil. To ensure all the petals are covered, you can fill the jar one inch above the top of the petals. Seal the jar tightly with its lid and place it in your pantry or basement food storage area. Let the jar sit for between two and eight weeks. During this time, the oil will leech the fragrance and healing properties from the petals.

After the allotted time has passed, strain the petals out of the jar using a cheese cloth, fine mesh strainer or a coffee filter and funnel. Pour the resulting oil into an oil bottle and cap. The oil can be used to enhance the flavour of foods and as a massage oil.

Warnings

There are no known side effects from using roses or rose petals as a herbal remedy. However, if you are allergic to roses, you should not use any herbal remedies containing roses or rose petals.

12. Toothpaste - Making your own

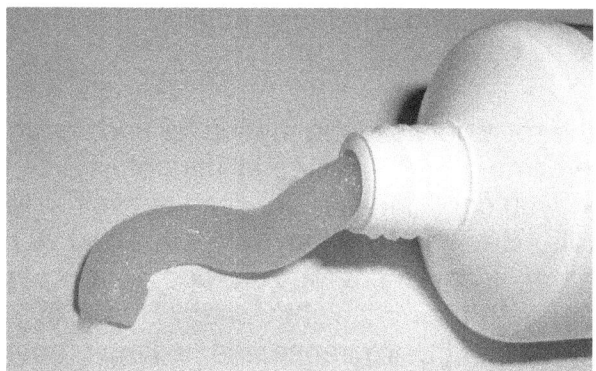

Origins

Toothpaste was first invented in the early 1900s. The first available flavour was cherry, and it was sold in small porcelain jars that required dipping the toothbrush into the paste. It was even available in the rooms of the Titanic for the guests and crew.

Today, toothpaste comes in metal tubes in a variety of mint flavours and cherry is no longer an option.

Ailments

Toothpaste whitens teeth and keeps teeth and guns clean, but most people do not know that it also helps with dry skin and pimples.

How It's Used

To use for dry skin and pimples, simply apply a small about of toothpaste to your hands and wash your face or the affected area just as you would with soap and water. The toothpaste will thoroughly clean and disinfect the pimple and the mint will reduce the redness and swelling. The slight abrasiveness of the toothpaste will remove dead and dry skin cells, leaving your face both looking and feeling clean and tingly. It's also a good way to cool down after a hot day or a rigorous workout.

Basic Toothpaste

This simple toothpaste will clean and whiten your teeth at a fraction of the cost of commercially available toothpastes.

Ingredients

Baking Soda
Water

Put a few tablespoons of baking soda in a dish. Rinse your toothbrush with water and dip it into the baking soda. Use it just as you would normal toothpaste. The baking soda will not foam. Toothpaste does not need to foam in order to get your teeth clean and disinfected, and it's healthier for your mouth and body. Commercially prepared toothpastes contain sulphates. The baking soda is slightly abrasive and will remove all the debris and plaque from your teeth. With repeated use, it can even remove stains and help whiten teeth.

Normal Toothpaste

Ingredients

1/2 Cup Baking Soda
2 Tablespoons Plus More Distilled water Or Hydrogen Peroxide
1 to 2 Teaspoons Mint extract
Food Processor
Small Glass Jar with A Lid

In a food processor, add the baking soda and pulse a few times until it is extra fine. Add two tablespoons of distilled water or peroxide and the mint extract. Pulse the machine again. If the mixture it too dry, add another tablespoon of water and pulse again. Do this until your toothpaste has the desired consistency.

Put the paste in a glass jar and seal tightly with the lid. A plastic bottle will not work for toothpaste as it will continuously dry out, and you will have to rehydrate it, which can be a hassle.

This recipe can be used as a toothpaste and as an acne remedy. Just make sure to add lots of mint extract.

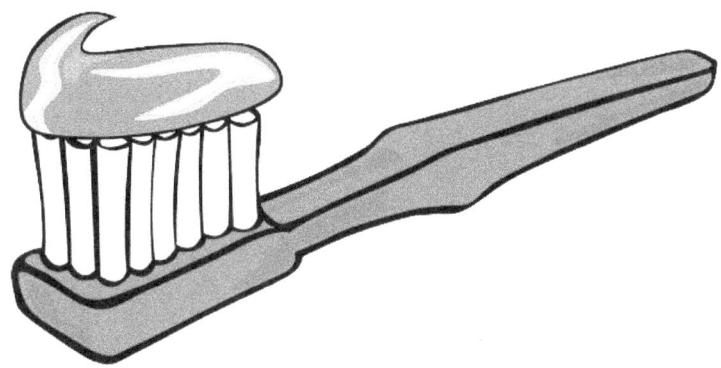

Advanced Toothpaste

Ingredients

1/2 Cup Baking Soda
2 Tablespoons Plus More Distilled water Or Hydrogen Peroxide
1 Tablespoon Coconut Oil
1/2 Teaspoon Coarse Salt or Sea Salt
1 Teaspoon Artificial Sugar
1 to 2 Teaspoons Mint extract
Food Processor
Small Glass Jar with A Lid

Put the baking soda and salt in the food processor and pulse until the grains are very fine. This is especially important for the salt. Large grains of salt can cause pain and damage your gums. Add the coconut oil, artificial sugar, water and mint extract and pulse. If the mixture is too dry, add a few more drops of water and continue to pulse until the paste is the right consistency. The coconut oil will keep the paste from drying out and help it maintain the desired consistency. Put the paste in an airtight glass jar and seal with a lid. It is now ready to be used on your teeth and face.

The salt and sugar can be omitted from the recipe.

Warnings

There are no side effects from using this toothpaste. It contains all-natural ingredients.

13. General Herbal Remedy Warnings

Vitamins and minerals purchased from vitamin stores in some countries are not regulated by the FDA. This means that each bottle could contain different amounts of the desired product. To keep your recipes consistent, buy the same brand. If you are taking OTC or prescription medications, make sure to schedule an appointment with your general practitioner and talk to a pharmacist. Some herbal remedies can react with some medications and cause unwanted side effects.

14. Special Offer & Links

Well, firstly I hope you enjoyed the book. Yet again, I had great fun writing it with my Grandma's help. I think this will be the last in the series. Well, at least until I can get Grandma to help out with some more anyway.

Special Offer

If you would like to receive a **free book** of any of the other Grandma's book series, please write a **review on Amazon** of the book and email me at ahsmithers@gmail.com and I will happily send you a copy of a free book of your choice.

Get All The Books In The Series:
Anton Smithers Books

The Grandma Series:-

Grandma's Herbal remedies

Grandma's Herbal Remedies – The Secret Recipes

Grandma's Guide to raising Backyard Chickens

New Technology – New Money Series

Everything you need to know about buying, selling and investing in BITCOIN

The 3D Printing revolution – Licence to Print Money

Health & Natural living

The amazing benefits of Coconut oil – Secret of the tropics

The amazing benefits of Tamanu Oil – secret of the south pacific

Top 10 Psoriasis Treatments

Top 10 Diets of all time

COMING SOOON – Grandma's Herb Garden Secrets